Alzheimer's Legacy Guide: A Financial Guide for Alzheimer's Patients and Caregivers

Helping Alzheimer's patients avoid the many hidden consequences of selecting the wrong beneficiaries for their life insurance policies, annuities and retirement accounts

Dennis M. Postema

The information contained herein is published for general purposes only. It is not meant to serve as an individual, personalized investment guide or suggestion. Additionally, the information used for samples does not guarantee the return that individual investors will receive. All information is based on tax codes and regulatory guidelines at the time of writing.

For personal investment advice, please call (419) 782-2500.

Agency edition: March 2014

Table of Contents

About the Author

Dennis M. Postema, RFC, is a successful entrepreneur, best-selling author, coach, speaker and registered financial consultant. He is the founder of MotivationandSuccess.com, StoriesofPerseverance.org, FinancingYourLife.com and TheRetirementInstitute.org.

Over the past 12 years, Dennis has taught clients, agents and associates how to find motivation and ascend psychological barriers to achieve success. His dedication to improving lives has led him to work with renowned motivational and self-help industry heavyweights, such as Jack Canfield and Brian Tracy.

Dennis' personal experience with tragedy, life-changing surgeries and health issues has given him a unique perspective on what it means to achieve success and what's really standing in the way of it. He channels that perspective into educational and motivational books and programs in the topics of finance, perseverance, success and business.

His focus on helping clients, rather than simply selling products, landed him on the cover of *Agents Sales Journal* (Senior Market Edition) in 2011.

In 2012, he was a recipient of the 10 Under 40 Award given by the Defiance Chamber of Commerce. He was also awarded the 2013 Distinguished Alumni Award from his alma mater, Northwest State Community College, for his success in the industry and community. His contribution to Jack Canfield's book, *Dare to Succeed*, earned him an Editor's Choice award.

Dedication

To my better half, my wife Jen; you're my best friend and full support system. Thank you for putting up with me during all of my projects that make our schedules crazy.

To my family, friends and team who make all that I do possible.

Finally, to all those people out there who have been part of a nightmare beneficiary situation or who currently are, but don't even know it. It's my hope that this book will give you unbiased advice that can truly educate you and wake you up before the nightmare begins...

Disclaimer

All information provided in this text has been researched and is accurate and complete to the best of the authors' knowledge. The authors are not responsible for any errors or omissions, and there is no guarantee of completeness, accuracy or timeliness regarding the information provided throughout this book.

You may use this information however you feel necessary, but you assume full responsibility for any potential loss that may occur from its use. Dennis M. Postema will not be liable for any direct, indirect, consequential, special, incidental, punitive or other damages whatsoever. Under no circumstance will Dennis M. Postema, related partnerships, corporations or other direct relationships of the author be held liable to you or anyone else for any information relied upon by you from this text. You assume full risk and responsibility for how you use the information provided herein.

All information in this book was accurate at the time of publication, and may change at any time. Modifications in the market, laws or other circumstances that arise may cause these facts to change. The information provided throughout this book may not be assumed to be correct at all times. Individual and global economic changes can cause the results herein to vary at any time. All decisions made due to information provided in this book are the sole responsibility of the reader.

Author's Note

One of the saddest situations our agency encounters is what we call the "Beneficiary Nightmare Scenario." It may sound lighthearted and, when caught in time, we can all poke fun at it. Unfortunately, it's often not until the choices that created the foundation for the nightmare are permanent that we find out about it—and at that point, there's nothing we can do to fix it.

The improper appointment of beneficiaries, wrong paperwork and ignorance of the complexities of tax and estate planning have led many people down the beneficiary nightmare path. This book was designed to be your lantern in the dark cavern of the nightmare. With it, you may light your path, avoid the monsters under the bed and design the ultimate estate plan to protect your loved ones after your passing while ensuring that the majority of your assets are transferred to the generations of family you leave behind—not the IRS.

No book is a substitute for a good advisor or estate planner. We strongly suggest that you take what you learn and, armed with that information, find an advisor who can help you create a plan of action that is thorough and attacks beneficiary and estate planning from all angles. Then get a good night's sleep, one that's totally nightmare-free.

Introduction

When asked to name a beneficiary on your life insurance policy, annuity or retirement account, the answer may seem like a no-brainer. Maybe you want your heirs—your family—to inherit your legacy. Or, maybe you want a charity to reap the benefit of your hard work. Or maybe you think it's best just to name your estate.

The financial reality of beneficiary appointment, however, is much more complex. There could be advantages and disadvantages to naming certain individuals or entities as the beneficiary of an account or policy. There could even be more efficient ways to accomplish what you have planned for the legacy you leave behind. Frankly, the wrong beneficiary choice could actually create a nightmare for your legacy and your heirs.

The goal of *Alzheimer's Legacy Guide: A Financial Guide for Alzheimer's Patients and Caregivers* is to give you an easy-to-use reference tool that makes efficient estate planning even simpler for newly diagnosed Alzheimer's patients and their caregivers. Each section starts with some real, albeit nightmarish, scenarios. Then you'll get the lowdown on what may seem like routine beneficiary election options and learn some strategies you may not have heard about before—all of which will help you avoid the nightmare scenario.

At the end of the book, there are worksheets, forms and letter templates to help you capitalize on the lessons you take from this book.

Preface: Special Planning for Those with Alzheimer's

In the early 1900s, German psychiatrist and neuropathologist Alois Alzheimer changed the world when he found plaque buildup and clumps of filament in what should have been the empty space between nerve cells while studying a particular patient's brain cells after her death. It was these two substances that explained the patient's complaints of memory lapses, disorientation, not recognizing family members and loss of ability to communicate through language during her last years of life. Thankfully, Dr. Alzheimer noted that these symptoms were not consistent with her relatively young age or any known disorder. In so doing, he discovered the heartbreaking and confusing disease of Alzheimer's.

Despite its relatively limited treatment options, Alzheimer's isn't some obscure disorder that few people have heard of. In 2012, the Alzheimer's Association reported that one in eight people over the age of 65 and 50 percent of people over the age of 85 had the disease. In total, 5.4 million individuals were reported to have the disease in 2012. Over the next 40 years, the Association expects that number to grow to as many as 16 million.

A diagnosis of Alzheimer's is terrifying at any age. While the disease has few physical manifestations, the mental, emotional and psychological effects it has can be devastating. If you've spent your life working toward building a legacy to pass on to your heirs, you won't want a diagnosis of Alzheimer's, or any other disease, to sabotage your efforts. Unfortunately, the very nature of the disease can make legacy planning—and the actualization of that plan—extremely difficult to fulfill. Therefore, it is extremely important to have a specialized tool that addresses the specific challenges Alzheimer's patients and their families face when it comes to estate planning.

Safeguarding Savings

You can't leave a legacy behind if you have no money or property left upon your passing. If you aren't careful, the Alzheimer's disease can have many ways to undermine your budget and devastate your savings.

Long-Term Care Policies

One way Alzheimer's can create a legacy nightmare for you and your heirs is by ravaging your savings through the cost of care as the disease progresses. Sadly, a long-term care policy may not be approved once a diagnosis is final. However, if you've secured one in the past it will go a long way in preserving your assets while ensuring uncompromised care.

If you have an existing long-term care policy, you should review its benefits. Study its waiting periods, inflation adjustments, limits and so on so you understand what expense overlap may fall to you and plan accordingly. Be sure to communicate this to any caregivers in your family and give them a copy of the policy so they can get familiar with its benefits and exercise all your options as soon as necessary.

Bill Payment and Power of Attorney

Understanding the ways the disease's progression can affect your finances is important in developing methods to fight it. For example, you may begin having difficulty remembering to pay bills on time, which can result in late payments, penalties and—if it goes on long enough—liens against your property. To avoid this, consider naming a financial power of attorney immediately upon being diagnosed. That individual may then ensure your bills are paid, checks are deposited and your finances remain in good standing throughout the years. Once you appoint a power of attorney, be sure to send copies of the POA paperwork to your trustee, your bank, your insurers, your lenders, your credit card issuers and so on. Then, set up a bill payment and financial monitoring system with your chosen POA. The system should allow you to stay in the loop but also ensure your POA is watching over the activity to make certain timely payments are made in the correct amount.

The development of a monitoring system can be difficult for many because it means allowing another family member, friend or trusted associate have an up-close glimpse of your personal financial position. It is, however, vital you take this step. It's also a good idea to discuss your future plans for retirement account distributions with the individual as well as how you intend to adjust your budget and spending through the years. Although it may be stressful, doing so will ensure your overarching financial plans are carried out no matter what.

Protection from Those Who'd Take Advantage

Alzheimer's mercilessly attacks your ability to reason. For many, this means an inability to remain focused when it comes to the long-term goals they once had for their money. Sadly, there are many individuals who would take advantage of a sufferer's declining mental state. Tragic stories abound about the elderly—including those who suffer other dementia and maladies—being swindled by friends, family members and strangers. Because Alzheimer's is a progressive disease, you may be fine and focused most days after diagnosis but will eventually, gradually begin declining and lose sight of your original priorities. If the wrong person sees this progression, it offers the perfect opportunity for them to step in and take advantage. It's impossible to know how quickly this could happen or when it will begin; therefore, it is very dangerous to put off planning preventative measures.

No one in your family can know you're being swindled unless they have a handle on both your finances and ultimate objectives. Appointing a power of attorney and discussing your goals and objectives with him or her allows you to give an individual some power to recognize and stop any mishandling of your finances quickly upon discovery.

Another way to combat this is by creating an irrevocable trust. With an irrevocable trust, the decisions you make for the future of your money are not revocable. So, if someone tries to take advantage of your disease or you simply begin making unhealthy decisions, you will be prevented from finalizing them. This is, however, a binding move and not something that should be taken lightly. Additionally, it may be a good idea to consider a third party or institution as the trustee of the trust. That way, you never have to question the motives of your family members which can help maintain the relationships.

Even if you don't want to appoint anyone as a power of attorney immediately upon being diagnosed and you aren't comfortable with the idea of an irrevocable trust, consider sharing information with a few family members who you trust so they can watch over you as the years go by. Should any of them suspect you're being taken advantage of they can file for guardianship or conservatorship and obtain a freeze order for your assets.

Changing Priorities after Diagnosis

Sometimes, after an individual has been diagnosed with an incurable disease, their estate planning priorities change. Instead of leaving everything to their family, they may decide they want all or a portion of their estate to go to a foundation to help find a cure for the disease they have.

There are many ways one can donate all or some of his or her property to an Alzheimer's research foundation:

- Set up an endowment: With an endowment, you have some control over how your gifted funds are used by the organization. Therefore, you can ensure the money is focused on the activities of the organization you think are most important. Endowments are generally made up of a principal amount that provides an ongoing income (such as through stock dividends); therefore, they can also provide valuable long-term funding.

- Charitable remainder trust: On page 61, CRTs are discussed in detail, but basically, they allow a donor to purchase an income-generating annuity with the funds they plan to donate to the organization while enjoying a tax deduction for the donation. The income payments are made to the donor and the charity receives the principal upon the owner's death.

- Assigning a life insurance death benefit: One can always change the beneficiary of a life insurance policy or an annuity with a death benefit rider to an organization focused on Alzheimer's research.

- Leaving some or all of your retirement account balances: Check with your IRA custodian and/or benefits administrator to see if you can change your 401(k) and other retirement plan account beneficiaries to the organization. Before you do, be sure to read Chapter 2 to understand how they will be able to access the money once you pass away.

- Will or trust: When you have a revocable trust, you can update your trust documents to allow the chosen institution to receive part or all of your estate's proceeds. Likewise, you can update your will the same way. It is extremely important, if you have complex instructions with multiple beneficiaries besides the organization, that your official, witnessed documents are specific as to exactly what you want going to whom. Don't be afraid to list out individual objects, amounts and percentages for each beneficiary as well as what you want to happen in the event a personal beneficiary predeceases you. For more information, read about per stirpes and per capita on page 33.

No matter how you decide to design your estate plan, consider sharing all of your account, policy and other important records with the executor of your estate or trustee of your trust. Doing so will ensure the individual has access to your will, trust documents, life insurance policy, retirement accounts and other parts of your legacy. This will guarantee proper access and distribution after your death.

If you've made any final expense plans, such as funeral arrangements, be sure to share those with a trusted individual or the executor of your estate.

Chapter 1: Life Insurance

The goal of a life insurance policy is to provide funds to beneficiaries for various needs. The funds may be for college tuition expenses, lifestyle preservation, a supplement for a surviving spouse's retirement savings, debt repayment, burial expenses—the list goes on and on.

For families dealing with a diagnosis of Alzheimer's or dementia, not only can life insurance offer a way to protect the legacy you want to leave to heirs, the cash value growth can also create a means of additional funding to pay for expensive treatment and care. In 2013, RAND Corp. announced its findings that the cost of providing care to someone with dementia was about $42,000 per year. This is a difficult financial burden for any family, but one that a cash value life insurance policy can help carry.

You may think the only consideration in terms of beneficiary election for your life insurance policy is the future purpose of the death benefit, but there is more to it than that.

Life Insurance Nightmare #1

There is nothing you want more than for your wife, Amy, to move on with her life after you pass. Then, when Amy remarries five years after your death, she thinks of you and knows you would give your blessing.

What Amy doesn't consider, and what you didn't realize when you left Amy as your primary beneficiary on your life insurance policy, is that your death benefit would end up in her second husband's hands after her death.

This prevents your children from receiving the remainder of your death benefit until, upon Husband Number 2's death, it is split amongst your children and his children from a prior marriage.

Life Insurance Nightmare #2

When your son Jack was born, you took out a $100,000 life insurance policy and named your wife as the primary beneficiary and your son as the contingent. You believed it was more than likely your wife would end up with the benefit and that she would use it to help secure the lifestyle she and Jack were used to. She may even use some of the death benefit toward Jack's college savings.

Unfortunately, just after Jack's 19th birthday, both you and your wife perish in a car accident. At 19, Jack is more responsible than some his age, but he is still lured by the appeal of hot cars, big TVs, and expensive Smartphone contracts. Within a year, the death benefit he gained as your contingent beneficiary is gone and all he has to show for it is an expensive car and some computer equipment.

Life Insurance Nightmare #3

When you took out your $500,000 life insurance policy, there was no question you would name your husband, Henry, the beneficiary. During your happy 25-year marriage, you and Henry had four children who went on to have a total of 15 grandchildren. Over the years, your family has remained close and you enjoy spending time together during holidays and vacations. As you look around at your children and grandchildren during your most recent get-together, you smile as you think of your life insurance policy death benefit and how, after you pass on, it will go to Henry and then, after he passes, will go toward enriching the lives of your children and grandchildren.

The truth after you pass away, however, is much less gratifying. Your $500,000 death benefit does go to Henry, but when Henry passes away, the funds are considered part of his estate. Now, before his estate can pass on to your children and grandchildren, they must pay a 35 percent tax on your death benefit and all other assets. While the net amount they receive still helps pay for college tuition expenses, your legacy doesn't do nearly as much as you'd hoped.

Beneficiary Basics

In a life insurance policy, beneficiaries are the named individuals or entities that will be paid your death benefit by your life insurance company.

Primary Beneficiaries

The individuals you most want to receive your death benefit will be listed as your primary beneficiaries. You can name more than one and can assign a percentage of the benefit for each to receive.

Contingent Beneficiaries

If your primary beneficiaries predecease you, your contingent beneficiaries will receive your death benefit in the increments you designate. For exceptions, see per stirpes and per capita designations beginning on page 32. If you name a trust as your primary beneficiary, there is no need to name a contingent since an entity never dies and has its own contingency plan.

Naming a Spouse or Significant Other as Beneficiary

When you have no children or very young children, your first instinct is likely to name your spouse or significant other as beneficiary. As the recipient of your death benefit, your spouse will be able to continue supporting your family even after losing your income. They will be able to contribute to retirement and college saving accounts, pay for burial and funeral expenses, and possibly even pay off debt.

Increasing Your Spouse's Taxable Estate

Once your spouse receives your death benefit, the money will become part of his or her taxable estate when he or she passes away. This can reduce the effectiveness of your death benefit, as it would then be subject to estate taxes.

If your spouse puts the death benefit funds to use or takes estate planning measures, such as investing in a grantor-retained annuity trust (GRAT), irrevocable trust, family limited partnership, gifts it to a charity, or invests in a limited-pay or single-premium whole life insurance policy, it could reduce or remove the estate tax liability.

Issues of Significant Others

The underwriters who review your application for life insurance coverage want to make sure there is an insurable interest, an emotional or financial loss that will be experienced upon your death, by the individual you name as beneficiary. If you are not married and wish to name your significant other, you can do so; just specify on the application that the individual is your partner or significant other in order to explain the insurable interest.

Any spouse or significant other can remarry or comingle assets with another individual after your death, and it's important to consider how this makes you feel about your death benefit proceeds since they could end up going to a new spouse or mate after your death. A trust (discussed in more detail on page 36) can prevent this and keep your legacy allocated only to your chosen heirs.

Medicaid and Other Assistance

When naming a spouse the beneficiary of your life insurance policy, the death benefit proceeds could also increase their assets and reduce their ability to qualify for financial assistance programs such as Medicaid. This could mean you'd be better served naming a trust or your children as the beneficiary so your spouse can still get the benefits he or she needs without your death benefit proceeds becoming a sacrificial lamb to their expenses.

Naming Children as Beneficiaries

It can seem very natural to name your children as beneficiaries to your life insurance policy, especially if you plan for the benefit to provide them with a means to pay college tuition expenses, wedding costs, a new home down payment or just as a general investment in their future. Before writing their names on the application as beneficiaries, however, you must decide whether to split the benefit equally among them or to favor one over another. Also, if some of them are young, you may decide it is better to appoint a trust as the beneficiary, and then give the trust instructions for distribution once the child has reached a certain age or taken a particular path in life, such as enrolling in college.

Even when naming multiple children as the beneficiaries of your policy, you must still choose a contingent beneficiary, unless you decide to have the benefits distributed *per stirpes* or *per capita*—a selection that must be noted on your beneficiary election. Per stirpes distributes benefits by family branches whereas per capita focuses on equal distribution by generation.

Additional Considerations

- *If you have an existing, court-required prenuptial, postnuptial or divorce agreement, then you may not have any flexibility in naming beneficiaries.*

- *If your spouse or significant other has a history of financial mismanagement, then you may wish to proceed to the trust section and discover how naming a trust the beneficiary can give you more control over how benefits are spent.*

Per Stirpes

A per stirpes distribution allows the second and, in some cases, future generation branches of a deceased primary beneficiary to receive a percentage of the death benefit. In this arrangement, the entire portion of the benefit assigned to the deceased individual is passed on to his or her survivors to split amongst themselves.

Per Capita

If you choose a per capita distribution and one or more of your beneficiaries predecease you, then the death benefit is divided into equal portions for all of the living second-generation family members of the deceased primary beneficiary.

Per Stirpes Example

Mary had three children whom she named beneficiary of her life insurance policy. She left one-third of the death benefit to each of them. Sadly, two of the children predecease her. One of them, Mark, left behind two children of his own and the other, Sharon, left behind one. Sharon's one-third of the death benefit will pass on to her child, just as Mark's will pass on to his—but while Sharon's child has no one to split it with, Mark's children will have to split his portion. Sally, the still-living child, will also get her third.

Per Capita Example

As in the example above, Mary had three children whom she named beneficiary of her life insurance policy. She left one-third of the death benefit to each of them. Sadly, two of the children predecease her. One of them, Mark, left behind two children of his own and the other, Sharon, left behind one. In a per capita arrangement, the still-living child, Sally, will receive one-third of the death benefit. The remaining two-thirds will be split evenly among both Sharon and Mark's children.

Instances of Ownership and Taxes

Potential tax consequences are another important consideration when determining your beneficiary(ies). Many people believe life insurance proceeds are distributed completely tax-free, but that's not always the case. To ensure it is, one must properly plan beneficiary and ownership designation, a lesson usually imparted by an advisor, but often ignored.

> *When the beneficiary on your policy, be it your spouse, your child or another relative, is also the owner of the policy, then they have an ownership in the cash value that grows within the policy, which can be accessed before death. When this is the case, the payment of the death benefit may be considered a taxable income to the owner/beneficiary.*

If you need your beneficiary to have some control over your policy as you age, then instead of meaningful ownership, you can complete a power of attorney document. This allows the beneficiary—provided he or she is also the named power of attorney—a limited ability to manage your policy but won't give him an ownership interest in the cash value. Finally, there is always the option to appoint a trust as the owner, which we will discuss in detail later in this chapter.

Additional Considerations

- *Having an instance of ownership in your policy isn't the only way your beneficiaries could be taxed. Insurance companies allow beneficiaries to choose a method of payout for the death benefit. If they choose to have the benefit paid out in one lump sum, and they are not an owner, then that death benefit should not be subject to federal estate taxes. If they instead opt for installment payments, then the principal death benefit will earn interest while the insurance company holds it. When this earned interest is paid out with the installments, the beneficiary may have to pay taxes on the additional gain.*

- *If your beneficiary invests the death benefit in an asset that experiences a gain, such as a stock, mutual fund or piece of real estate, then when they sell the asset, it could be subject to long- or short-term capital gains taxes.*

Naming an Estate as Beneficiary

In order to avoid family rivalry or fighting or in an effort to make estate management easier, many people decide to name their estate as the beneficiary of their life insurance policy. *This decision could hurt your heirs more than you think*, because when an estate is named beneficiary of a life insurance policy, the death benefit proceeds are added to the gross estate for federal estate tax purposes. With the estate exemption falling in 2013, this can result in a very harmful consequence to your legacy.

Did You Know?

---

* *If you leave the beneficiary election blank on your application, most insurance companies will record your estate as your beneficiary.*

A Trust as Beneficiary

Many of the challenges associated with naming one or more individuals as the beneficiary of your life insurance policy can be avoided when you name a trust, such as a revocable or irrevocable life insurance trust (ILIT), the owner and beneficiary.

A trust is a legal agreement in which the grantor (the person who creates the trust) assigns assets to the trust for the benefit of a beneficiary. The beneficiary (or beneficiaries) can be himself/herself or other individuals and entities. The trust then appoints a trustee to manage the assets, pay taxes and execute the directives within the trust document.

The trust document can specify when a beneficiary is to receive an asset, under what conditions and how often. Trusts can be created to pay out an income made on principal assets or can pay out principal and income over many years. It's a very personal document and plan that allows an unparalleled amount of control over assets before and after your death.

Having your life insurance policy inside a trust cannot only help you avoid many of the taxation issues that could be impacted by your beneficiary selection, but it also gives you an unparalleled level of control over the distribution of your assets.

Within the trust documents, you can determine who receives death benefit proceeds as well as when. If you have young children, this can help ensure they don't receive a large sum of money before they are emotionally equipped to handle it properly. If you have a spouse who is not disciplined in managing money, the trust can make regular payments to him or her so you don't have to worry about any spendthrift tendencies.

Finally, there is the assurance that if your spouse remarries or your significant other comingles assets with another individual after your death, your legacy will still get to the people you wanted it to rather than to the heirs of the new mate.

In addition, because there is no personal beneficiary instance of ownership in the life insurance policy, the cash values that accumulate within the policy can generally be kept safe from creditors through various laws in the owner and beneficiary's state of residence.

Assets inside the trust which are allowed to grow and earn additional income can create tax consequences for the trust, so it's best to have a third-party fiduciary who understands the tax and management responsibilities of being a trustee.

Did You Know?

- *If you create the wrong kind of trust, your assets may not be safe from creditors after all. Talk to an advisor about the pros and cons of all the various trust options before you make a decision.*

- *If you are the parent of a child with special needs, a Special Needs Trust will help ensure their trust payments do not remove their government aid eligibility.*

Naming a Charity or Church as Beneficiary

If you are charitably inclined, then you always maintain the option of naming a charity or church as the beneficiary of your life insurance policy. You can name any charity or religious organization you wish, and there are no estate tax ramifications in doing so.

There are more tax-efficient ways to give money to charity through a life insurance policy that allow you to enjoy a benefit while you are still living, such as by gifting or donating the policy itself to a qualified charity. This can allow you some income tax deductions. However, this step cannot be reversed and is a little more complex than simply naming a charity the beneficiary of your life insurance policy.

When you name a charity as your beneficiary, you have no obligation to tell the charity or your family that you have done so. Further, you can always change your mind later and submit the necessary paperwork to rename your beneficiary. It is important, however, that you leave notification instructions somewhere, such as in your will, to ensure the charity does eventually find out about your policy and submit the requisite claim forms.

Naming a Funeral Home or Creditor as Beneficiary

Some individuals, especially those with term insurance policies, consider naming funeral homes or creditors as their life insurance beneficiaries, but this can be a bad idea.

If the money spent at the funeral home is less than your death benefit, it can be difficult and time consuming for your family to get a refund. While all your other assets may be stuck in probate or liquidated by creditors, this can put your family in a tough spot.

Funeral Homes

When naming a funeral home the beneficiary of a policy, you ensure your relatives bear no burden for your funeral and burial expenses. However, you also take away the flexibility they might have had in deciding the best way to pay for the benefits. You also encourage the funeral home to push for a funeral that costs whatever your death benefit is—when your children and spouse might have more pressing issues for that money.

Creditors

It is common for new homeowners to buy term life insurance and name their lender as the beneficiary of the policy. If you purchased a decreasing term policy with a death benefit that is designed to decrease over time along with your mortgage balance, then this can be a good strategy. If you choose to do this, then you should also have separate life insurance benefits or assets available to your family that will not be tied up in probate.

If all you have is the term policy, then leaving your spouse, significant other or children as beneficiary allows them to use the proceeds for more pressing matters that come up after your death. Then, when the estate is settled, they can use other assets to pay off the mortgage.

To-Do List

- Decide how you want your death benefits used and which members of your friends and family you want to benefit from them.

- Use the flow chart on page 43 to help determine how to best structure your life insurance death benefit elections.

- Set up any trust plan you think will help preserve your assets and ensure their proper allocation. Meeting with an attorney prior to putting plans in writing is always recommended.

- Consider any tax consequences or creditor action your family may face after your death and secure additional life insurance benefits to compensate.

- Fill out the appropriate insurance company forms to make the relevant beneficiary changes. You can also use the form letter in Chapter 6.

- Decide how to tell your family about your life insurance policy(ies) and how much information you'll give them. You can remain vague, but it's important they have instructions about what to do after your death in order to get the benefits.

Flow Chart

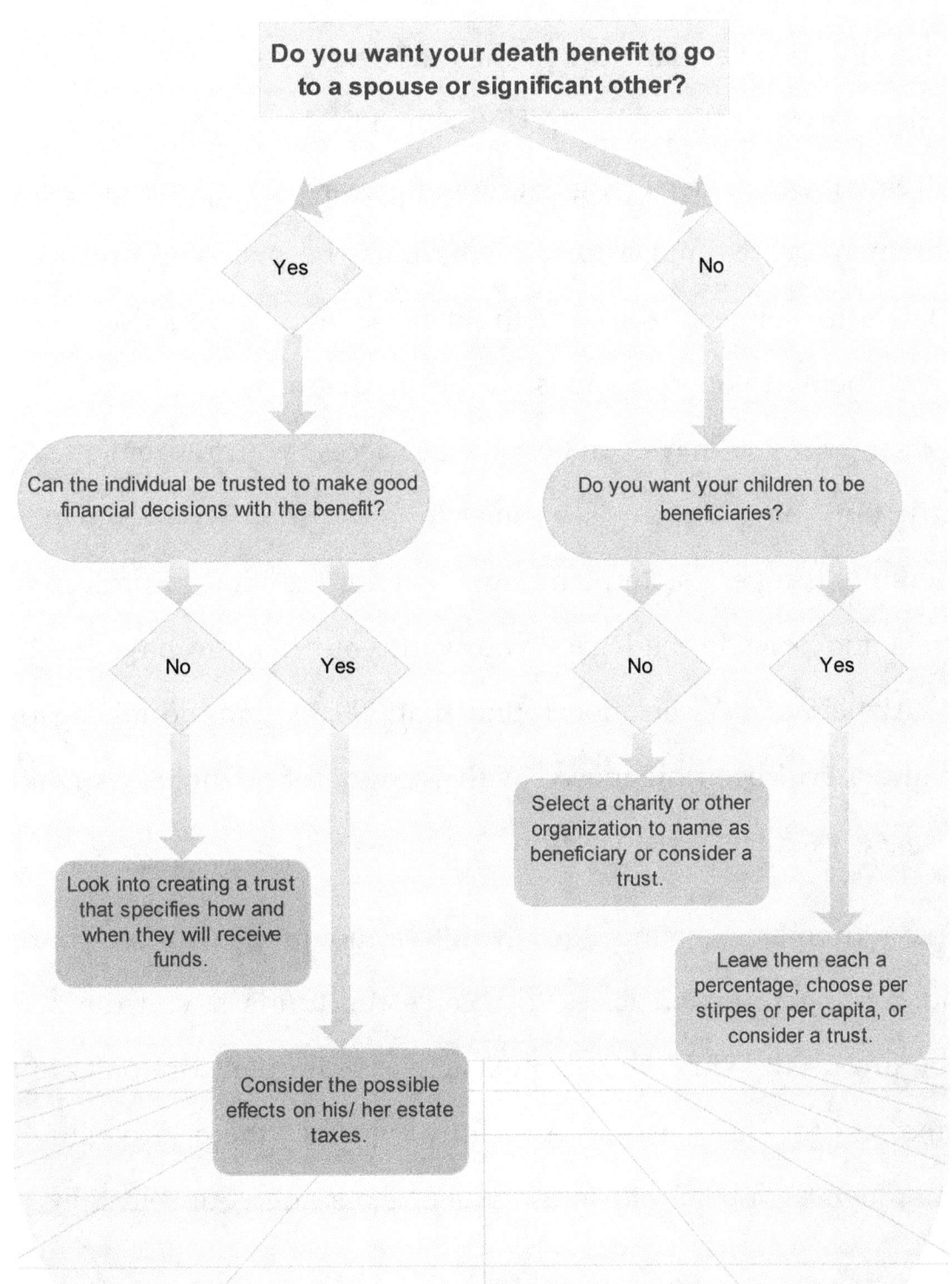

Chapter 2: Retirement Accounts

Generally, people plan to use their retirement savings to fund the golden years of their lives. Unfortunately, not everyone reaches retirement age or lives long enough afterward to deplete their saved retirement assets, and arrangements must be made in advance for what is to happen to your retirement savings if you don't get to spend them. If you or a spouse has been diagnosed with early-onset Alzheimer's, you may even be forced to access your retirement funds early and have much less time to save than you anticipated. Therefore, proper estate planning is even more vital to protect your assets and provide the legacy you want your heirs to have. In 2012, the Alzheimer's Association found that 200,000 individuals aged 64 or under had been diagnosed with early-onset Alzheimer's making this a very serious consideration.

Most retirement accounts allow you to appoint one or more primary and contingent beneficiaries to receive the funds if you die before they are used. While your beneficiary appointment options are the same as for life insurance death benefits, there are different consequences you should consider before making your selections.

Required Minimum Distributions

One important fact to remember about retirement plans that will actually play a huge role in how beneficiaries are affected is the required minimum distribution (RMD). RMDs are mandatory, IRS-calculated distributions that must be taken from certain retirement accounts once the owner reaches age 70 (for some accounts) or 70.5. The amount is based on the owner's life expectancy, and many beneficiaries will be affected depending if the owner's death occurs before or after they begin taking RMDs.

Now that the basics are out of the way, let's look at three nightmare scenarios everyone will want to avoid when planning their legacies.

Retirement Nightmare #1

You've named each of your six children, who range in age from 20 to 40 years old, a beneficiary of your 401(k). Instead of assigning each a percentage of the assets left at the time of your death, you give them each a dollar amount. Unfortunately, this means they must all take distributions annually that are based on the life expectancy of the oldest beneficiary. Therefore, your youngest child must take out much more of her share than she can afford to in terms of taxes. In addition, because the distribution isn't being stretched out over her life, the account will be depleted well before she reaches retirement.

Retirement Nightmare #2

Unable to decide whom you should make the beneficiary of your retirement accounts, you've left the estate as beneficiary and will allow the executor to distribute assets. Unfortunately, because you died prior to age 70.5 and were not receiving required minimum distributions (RMDs), your retirement account assets must be paid out to your estate within five years. Therefore, your family has no option to further delay taxes on the assets. They must liquidate the account holdings in a possibly unfavorable investment climate, and future generations may be left out in the cold.

Retirement Nightmare #3

A retiree and his wife, each with high-balance 401(k)s from the company they both worked for, were in a fatal car accident just before retiring. They had each named the other as the beneficiary of their individual 401(k)s; however, since they passed away at the same time, their 401(k) balances normally would have gone to their contingent beneficiaries. Unfortunately, in this case, they hadn't named any.

Because of this seemingly minor oversight, the $450,000 cumulative balance had to be paid out to their children in a lump sum, raising each adult child's tax brackets that year. Had the couple named their children as contingent beneficiaries, they would have had the freedom to stretch the benefits, possibly even keeping them multigenerational, and would have had little to no effect on their tax brackets.

Children and Other Nonspouse Beneficiaries

Making your children or any other individual who is not your spouse the beneficiary of a 401(k), IRA, 403(b) or other retirement account can present the same types of problems it does with other assets.

Firstly, the individual may receive the funds before he or she is ready to handle them responsibly. Another concern when naming a nonspouse as the beneficiary of a retirement account is how the funds can be paid out after death. Nonspouse beneficiaries cannot roll assets into their own IRA in order to treat the assets as part of their personal retirement plan. Instead, if the death occurs *before* the accountholder's required minimum distributions (RMDs) begin; the beneficiary can take a lump sum or, if they decide not to, they must at least begin taking required annual minimum distributions based on their life expectancy.

If the accountholder's death occurs after he or she began taking RMDs, the nonspouse beneficiary's RMDs are based on the longer life expectancy—his or the deceased accountholder's.

With 401(k), 403(b) and 457 plans, the nonspouse beneficiary may be able to transfer the proceeds to another trustee who acts as the custodian to an inherited IRA. This is not something you can set up for them in advance, so it may be worth discussing the process with your attorney and the individual(s) named as beneficiary. Lastly, in some cases, such as with a 401(k), your spouse may need to sign a waiver in order for the funds to go to your children or another nonspouse beneficiary.

Multiple Beneficiaries

When naming more than one child or individual as the beneficiary of a retirement account, one must be careful to give each person a percentage rather than a dollar amount. When giving multiple beneficiaries a dollar sum, the accountholder locks all the beneficiaries into receiving an RMD based on the age of the oldest beneficiary, which could result in larger distributions than each beneficiary wants and, thus, a larger tax burden.

Instead, by assigning each beneficiary a percentage of the retirement account value, you can ensure that separate accounts are created after your death and that the RMD is based upon each individual beneficiary's life expectancy.

Did You Know?

---

* *You can specify per stirpes and per capita distribution of the account balance in the event of the death of your primary beneficiary(ies).*

Stretch IRA or Multi-Generational IRAs

There are many benefits to stretching out the distribution of retirement account assets after your death. The first you might think of is that the longer they stretch it out, the longer your heirs have to pay taxes. In addition, the longer they can stretch the payout, the more generations it can reach and the less likely it is to be included in your beneficiary's estate for estate tax purposes, unlike a lump-sum payment, which would be included.

The stretch IRA is not something special you need to buy, and there are no special forms to complete. It's simply created when you name a nonspouse beneficiary on your IRA.

Spouse as Beneficiary

Spouses who inherit IRAs and other retirement accounts have a couple of options. They can roll over the assets into their own IRA (assuming it is the same type of IRA as the one they inherited or, in the case of a 403(b) or 401(k), any kind of IRA). When they do this, the minimum distributions are not just based on their life expectancy, but on the Uniform Life Table. This allows for a more generous time period for payout since it's based on both the life expectancy of the IRA accountholder and a beneficiary up to 10 years younger than the accountholder. This makes for a great legacy planning maneuver and allows assets to grow tax-deferred (or, in a Roth IRA, tax-free) even longer.

Spouses may also decide to transfer both IRA and 401(k) assets into an inherited IRA. When this occurs, required minimum distributions are determined based only on the life expectancy of the spouse who inherited the assets, which loses them a little bit of the legacy planning and tax-deferral power discussed above.

If the spouse beneficiary is concerned about taking the assets due to tax or other reasons, they have the option of denying them so they pass over to the contingent beneficiary(ies).

In some cases, a spouse may also be permitted to leave the assets in their spouse's account, using his or her date of birth and life expectancy table information for minimum distribution requirements.

Estate as Beneficiary

When naming an estate as the beneficiary of your retirement account, you give much less flexibility to your heirs. Not only will the accounts need to go through probate, thereby restricting your heirs' access to them, but all the proceeds must be paid out within five years of your death. If it is a Traditional IRA and you were 70.5 or older when you died, then RMDs must be taken according to the schedule when you were alive. This can create major tax consequences and reduce the amount of time the funds can grow tax-deferred. In addition, it can force your executor to liquidate your underlying investments at a time when it may not be advantageous to do so.

If you want to avoid this, it's not enough just to leave the beneficiary form blank because often that will prompt a custodian to automatically make the estate the beneficiary. Instead, name one or more individuals.

Trust as Beneficiary

When you name a trust as the beneficiary of your retirement plans, within the trust document, you must make sure to name individual beneficiaries to whom the trust is to pay out benefits. If you don't, then your estate will be considered the default beneficiary. Therefore, all the assets will need to be distributed within five years of your death, which can create a messy tax situation for generations of your heirs and make them miss out on upside potential as your investments will need to be liquidated.

When you name individual beneficiaries inside your trust, assets can be paid out according to the life expectancy of the oldest beneficiary.

It's a foregone conclusion that every descendant you'll ever have will not have been born at the time of your death. If you want to make allowances in your trust for the payment of benefits to all your descendants (including those not yet born), you can do so. Payments will still be based on the age and life expectancy of the oldest current descendant.

Charity as Beneficiary

When you name a charity as the beneficiary of your retirement funds, your heirs will pay no estate taxes on the funds. Nor will they benefit from them except through the progress your chosen charity(ies) is able to create with the funds. The charity may take payment in a lump sum or, if they wish to defer it, may need to take the payments within five years (if you passed away before needing RMDs) or over your calculated life expectancy (if you passed away after you began receiving RMDs) which is based on life expectancy tables in the year of your death.

Charitable Remainder Annuity Trusts

The next section discusses the power of creating a Charitable Remainder Annuity Trust (CRAT) to donate funds to charity and enjoy a current tax deduction, all while receiving an income from the underlying annuity. You may also designate a CRAT as a beneficiary of your retirement account (certain accounts only) and allow your beneficiaries to receive income payments from the CRAT while avoiding estate taxes on the underlying retirement funds since they are designated to charity.

To-Do List

- Determine how you want your retirement assets utilized after your death and consider how payout restrictions (the five-year-rule, life expectancy and uniform life expectancy tables) can affect your wishes *and* the account balance since they lead to asset liquidation.

- Set up any trust plan you think will help preserve your assets and ensure their proper allocation. Name individuals as beneficiaries within the trust or your retirement assets may need to be paid out much quicker than you'd like.

- Consider the benefit to your heirs of allowing a CRAT to be the beneficiary of your IRA assets.

- Decide how to tell your family about your retirement accounts and how much information you'll give them. You can remain vague, but it's important they have instructions about what to do after your death in order to get the benefits and to anticipate how their lives may change.

- Make a list of all your retirement account numbers, plan administrators' phone numbers and addresses.

- Use the flow chart below to help determine how to best structure your beneficiary choices.

Flow Chart

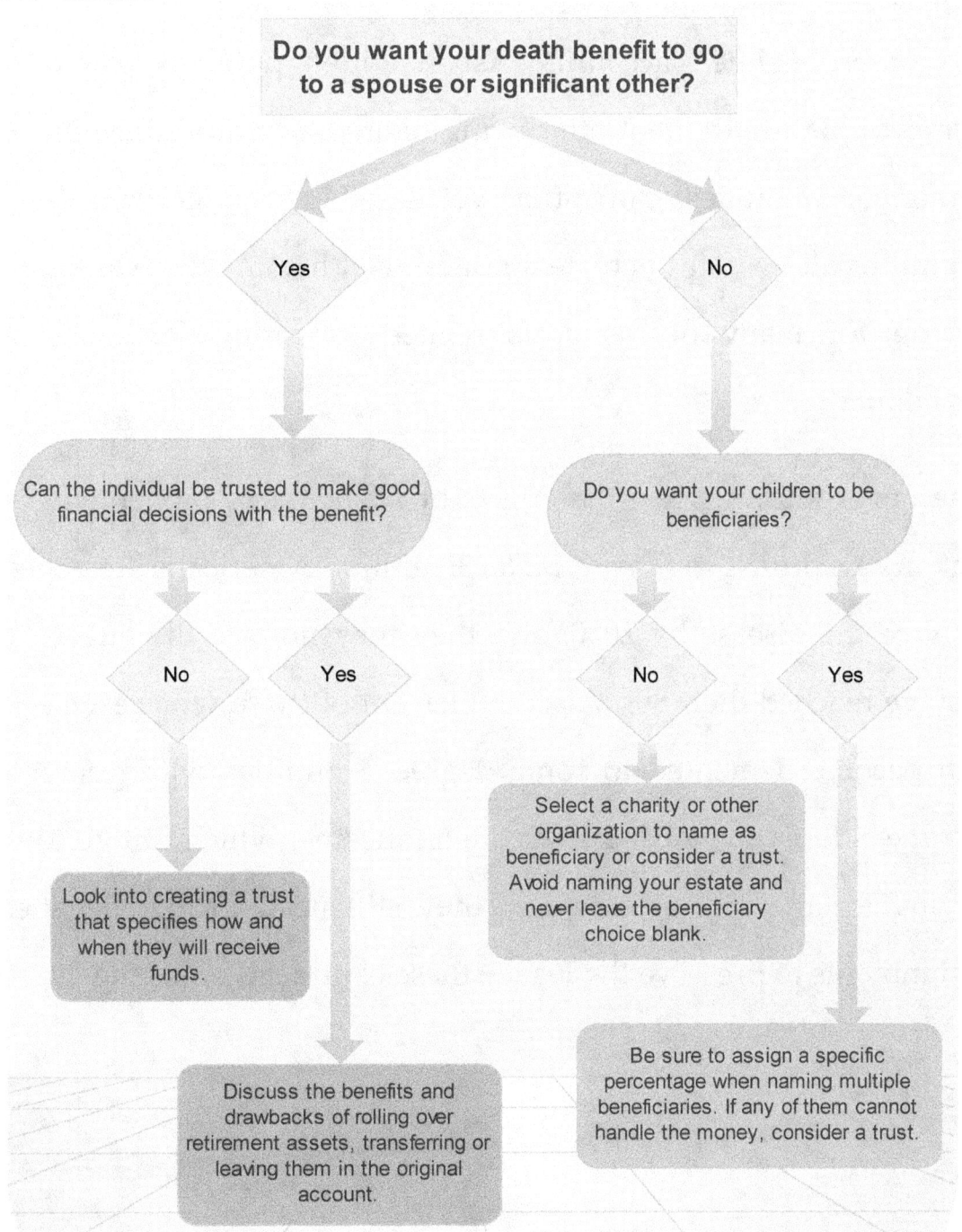

Chapter 3: Annuities

This section discusses the various options for naming an annuity beneficiary. This is only applicable for annuities held outside IRA and other qualified accounts. As an added note, for individuals trying to plan retirement after being diagnosed with Alzheimer's or dementia, annuities can offer yet another tremendous benefit. Annuities allow you to create a guaranteed income that can assist in paying for many of the costs related to caring for those with Alzheimer's.

One never knows when the effects of Alzheimer's or dementia will kick in. According to *Science Daily*, 30 million Americans are expected to have the disease by 2050, and they may not see the effects until they've reached their 80s. Also, 50 percent of those who reach age 85 will become demented to some degree. Annuities with guaranteed income riders can be used to create an income, which can go toward paying for the cost of care, but they still need proper beneficiary assignments to preserve the legacy these contracts can create.

Understanding Annuities

An annuity is a tool for ensuring an income after retirement or for creating a planned set of payments for a settlement or lottery winnings. Annuities go through an accumulation phase during which no payments are made and the principal is allowed to grow. If an annuity begins making income payments or is annuitized, the payout to beneficiaries after the death of the owner/annuitant can vary depending on the type of annuity involved:

- Straight life annuity: A straight life annuity without a death benefit rider will have no death benefit once it annuitizes.

- Period certain: A period certain annuity will continue making payments to the beneficiary for the remainder of the period certain.

- Joint and last survivor: A joint and last survivor annuity continues making payments as long as at least one of the annuitants is living. If the joint and last survivor annuity had a period certain and both annuitants pass away, the beneficiary can receive payments until the end of the period.

- Annuity with income rider: Some annuities offer the option of an income rider that can be utilized without being annuitized. This often leaves a full lump-sum death benefit still available to beneficiaries or an income payment should they choose this more flexible payment option.

Death Benefit Riders

Your agent may suggest you add a death benefit rider to your annuity. These riders can guarantee different benefits depending on the type of annuity you select. In a variable annuity, one with underlying subaccounts filled with investments subject to possible market losses, a death benefit rider can ensure your beneficiaries at least receive the principal contributed to the annuity. In a product such as an indexed annuity, the rider is guaranteed to grow interest on top of premiums paid in and can ensure your beneficiaries receive an amount equal to the highest recorded value for the annuity during a certain period of time or its full accumulated value.

Qualified versus Nonqualified

Another factor that influences some of the information about annuity beneficiary choices is whether the annuity is qualified or nonqualified. A qualified annuity is one that is purchased for retirement purposes and has special tax deferrals. A qualified annuity is often purchased inside an IRA or 401(k). When a qualified annuity is within a retirement account, the account's beneficiary elections take precedence.

A nonqualified annuity is one purchased without the tax benefits of a retirement account.

Annuitant, Owner and Beneficiary

Much like a life insurance policy, an annuity can have three distinct people involved. The first is the annuitant. This is the individual whose life the annuity death benefit is based on. It's also the individual to whom payments are made after the annuity annuitizes. The owner (or owners) of the annuity is the individual who contributes the principal to the annuity either in a lump sum or installments, and they name the annuity's beneficiary. The beneficiary, as you probably know by now, is the individual who receives death benefits through a death benefit rider and, when relevant, the full accumulated value of the annuity. The way the ownership and annuitant structure is designed on the annuity has a bearing on various aspects of the taxation and payments of annuity values to a beneficiary.

In a joint-owned annuity, the surviving owner immediately becomes the beneficiary and may need to now name new beneficiaries. However, joint-owned annuities, when the joint owner is a nonspouse, can introduce additional problems in terms of gift taxes and reducing the lifetime gift tax exemption which also reduces your estate tax exemption.

Annuity Nightmare #1

Your period certain annuity has another three years' worth of payments to make at the time of your death. Your daughter, as the annuity's beneficiary, will receive those payments.

Unfortunately, the payments will be included in her ordinary income for income tax purposes. Not only will this increase her tax liability, but the amount of the payment bumps up her income enough to make it so she can no longer contribute to her Roth IRA. She is also now subject to alternative minimum taxes.

Annuity Nightmare #2

Your annuity with death benefit rider pays out a $100,000 death benefit upon your passing. In 10 years, your spouse, the beneficiary, takes the lump sum and uses it to buy the dream home for her and her new spouse. Upon her death, her new spouse takes full ownership of the dream house and all her other assets, leaving your children and grandchildren with nothing.

Annuity Nightmare #3

You name your daughter, who is also the executor of your estate, the beneficiary of your annuity. Your wishes are for her to split the annuity benefit with her brother, your only other child. After your death she does as you wish, but because she was the named beneficiary and received the assets from the insurance company, she was taxed on all the interest. It's even possible she will be charged gift taxes if your distribution instructions were not in the will.

Children as Beneficiaries

Unlike a life insurance policy, death benefits paid out from an annuity may be taxed under the beneficiary's ordinary income tax rate except under certain trust arrangements and, in some cases, could be included in your estate for estate tax purposes. The proceeds will not, however, be subject to probate. There may be an additional premature distribution penalty imposed if the benefit is paid out to the child from a nonqualified annuity if the owner is not the deceased annuitant.

Your beneficiary will have a few common options, including the choice to take either a lump sum or annuitize the contract and take payments out of the annuity over a five-year period. If they choose the latter, it can help spread their tax liability into multiple years, but it's important to note that their tax liability may be extremely high and based on the original purchase value of the annuity rather than on a stepped-up basis (explained below). Any return of principal paid out from an annuitized benefit is not considered part of the income tax liability.

Finally, a child can choose to stretch the payout over the course of their life expectancy; however, not all annuity contracts allow this option. If yours does and your child chooses it, a required minimum distribution (RMD) will be calculated annually based on the amount of the annuity and the current age and life expectancy of the child.

Alzheimer's Legacy Guide: A Financial Guide for Alzheimer's Patients and Caregivers

---

> ### Understanding Basis and Step-Ups
>
> *When passing on assets, such as stocks to your heirs, the cost basis (or price you paid to buy the investment that is generally exempt from capital gains tax) receives a bump, or step-up, to current value, which helps reduce your beneficiary's capital gains tax liabilities upon the sale of the asset.*
>
> *Nonqualified annuities receive no step-up in basis, therefore beneficiary planning is that much more important.*

Spouse as Beneficiary

If you are the owner of your annuity and name your spouse as the beneficiary, your spouse will be permitted to take a full death benefit or step in as the annuity's owner upon your death. Your spouse can then allow the contract to accumulate and annuitize, thereby deferring income taxes on a nonqualified annuity.

A spouse who is under age 59.5 may face penalties of up to 10 percent if they decide to step in as the annuitant and take early withdrawals, so they may be better served by taking the death benefit.

Significant Other as Beneficiary

A significant other who is not considered a spouse in a common-law state is treated as any other nonspouse beneficiary. As such, they can choose a lump-sum payout, the five-year option or a stretch payout as described in the Children as Beneficiaries section.

Estate as Beneficiary

When naming an estate the beneficiary of an annuity you force your annuity death benefit, payments and proceeds to go through probate with your other assets. In addition, you ensure the funds will be considered as part of the estate for estate tax purposes.

Having the estate as the beneficiary also limits the number of distribution options your heirs can enjoy. Per the IRS, annuity death benefits with an estate as the beneficiary must be paid out within five years of the annuitant's death.

Currently, one of the major concerns with an estate as beneficiary is the insecurity surrounding the future of estate taxes. In 2012, the estate tax rate was 35 percent. In 2013, it rose to 40 percent—and who knows what increases the future will bring.

Did You Know?

- *The entire account value of an annuity that has not annuitized is included in estate value for estate tax purposes when the beneficiary is a spouse or nonspouse. If an annuity has annuitized, the value of the remaining payments may be added to the estate.*

- *As with life insurance, a blank annuity beneficiary will prompt payment to the estate.*

Trust as Beneficiary

If you've decided to retain ultimate control over the who, what, when, where and why of the distribution of your assets after your death, then you've probably created a trust. When you name a trust as the beneficiary of your annuity, assets can be paid to the trust in a lump sum or over the five years after your death.

Trusts can keep assets safe from creditors, apply more structure to how benefits are paid out and add some tax benefits for beneficiaries, but are not tax-free. Simple trusts are those that only make distributions of income earned rather than principal. They make these distributions during the year they are earned and only pay those distributions to noncharitable beneficiaries and may create higher personal tax consequences to the beneficiary as they pass the taxable income onto them. Complex trusts may have charitable beneficiaries and don't need to pay out income the year it's earned. They can pay out a portion of principal as well and may keep more of the tax burdens unto itself if it doesn't pay out income to beneficiaries.

If your trust is the owner of your annuity, then by default, it should also be the beneficiary. This ensures the beneficiary arrangements of the trust are not bypassed.

Charity or Other Nonprofit as Beneficiary

Naming a charity as the beneficiary of your annuity not only ensures your favorite nonprofit organization is enriched by your legacy, but it can also provide personal income and tax benefits while you are living.

This is done by creating a charitable remainder annuity trust (CRAT) which allows you to irrevocably gift the principal of your annuity—the total of your personal contributions—to your charity. Because you are gifting this during your lifetime, you receive a tax deduction (up to a certain percent of your adjusted gross income) for the donation, provided the charity is a qualified institution.

Since annuities create income for the annuitant, the income the annuity earns while in the CRAT is paid out to you. Therefore, you can use the annuity to help fund your retirement while still ensuring you leave a legacy to a cause that matters to you *and* get a tax deduction in the process. It is important to remember that taxes will be due on any income received from the CRAT.

Selecting a Charity

The ultimate goal in selecting a charity for your CRAT is to choose one that means something to you. It may be a charity dedicated to helping people with the same medical condition you or a loved one has, it may be a church, a school, or any number of other institutions or medical research projects. Ultimately, the chosen organization must be nonprofit [such as a registered 501(c)(3)] but can be either publicly or privately funded.

When determining your deduction for the donation, it's best to meet with a tax advisor. Generally, for publicly funded organizations such as churches and hospitals, one can deduct an amount that's up to 50 percent of their adjusted gross income (AGI). For private organizations, the deduction can be up to 30 percent of their AGI with a five-year carry forward for the excess. Lastly, the contribution must generally be made in the same tax year as the deduction is taken.

Telling Your Heirs

It's up to you whether you decide to tell your heirs about your decision to leave assets to charity or another nonprofit. As part of your estate planning measures, you may have decided to arm your heirs with complete knowledge of how your assets will be distributed, or you may have thought it best to let them find out after your death when your trustee and/or executor begins to distribute assets.

Ultimately, you must choose the method of disclosure you feel will work best for you and your family.

To-Do List

- Determine how you want your annuity balances and death benefits utilized after your death and consider how payout restrictions could affect that plan if you name certain individuals as beneficiaries or joint annuitants.

- Use the flow chart on the next page to help determine how to best structure your annuity owner, joint owner and death benefit.

- Set up any trust plan you think will help preserve your assets and ensure their proper allocation.

- Consider the benefit of a current tax deduction for charitable donations that doesn't interrupt your annuity's personal income stream.

- Complete the appropriate insurance company forms to make the relevant beneficiary changes on your annuity. You can also use the form letter in Chapter 6.

- Decide how you will tell your family about your annuity(ies) and how much information you'll give them. You can remain vague, but it's important they have instructions about what to do after your death in order to get the benefits and to anticipate how their lives may change.

Flow Chart

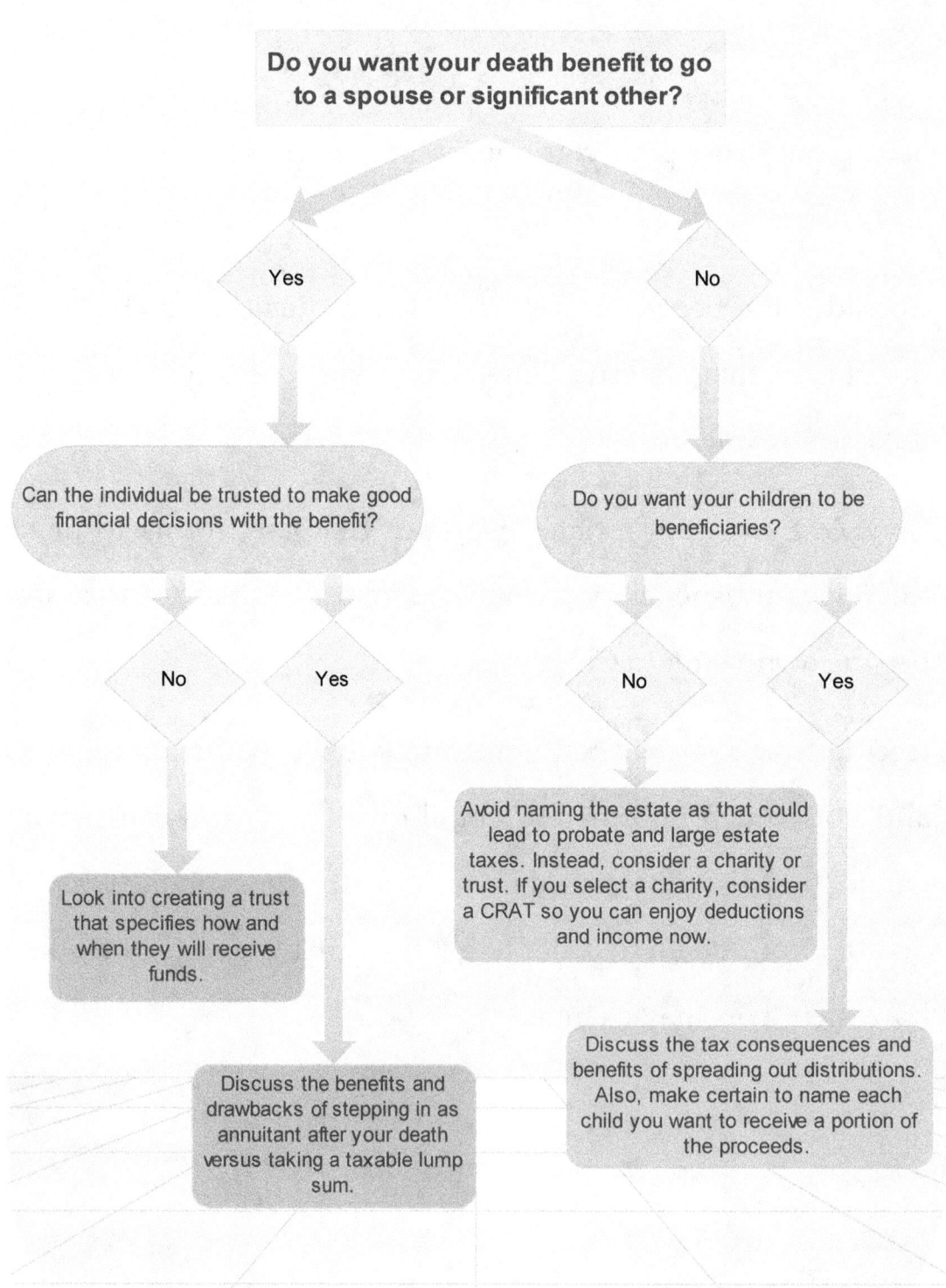

Chapter 4: A Note for Caregivers

There are many resources that discuss issues surrounding legacy planning and Alzheimer's disease, but the patients themselves aren't the only individuals affected by this diagnosis. In every family with an Alzheimer's sufferer, there are one or more caregivers who take some responsibility, either solely or with other family members, for the patient's finances and legacy.

Putting the Patient First

A caregiver's first priority will generally be to secure proper care for their loved one and make certain they can continue that care throughout the life of the afflicted individual. For some Alzheimer's patients, that could mean their assets are gradually depleted and there is little or no legacy to pass on to heirs. It's important to remember that this, in itself, is not a tragedy. The fact your loved one will be able to live out his or her life with dignity and good care is wonderful and a great way to create an intangible legacy of love and respect.

Caregivers who are responsible for the financial life of the patient might consider certain products, such as annuities with a guaranteed income, in order to help ensure the patient's savings are sufficient to secure that kind of care. First, however, they must assess the financial prospects by reviewing assets and making a budget with long-term spending projections.

Making a Budget

Handling the finances of a loved one suffering from Alzheimer's is much like handling your own finances. Therefore, as their guardian, power of attorney, trustee or representative payee, you should have a budget for income and expenses, and you should stick to it. Budgets are one of the few ways you can ensure the patient's savings last and readily show how you've been managing their finances should questions arise.

When creating the budget, consider the regular monthly income the individual receives from sources such as:

- Traditional IRAs (remember these distributions are taxable and the accounts have required minimum distributions that begin at age 70.5)

- Roth IRAs

- Social Security

- Pensions

- Veteran's benefits

- Insurance and annuity payments

Next, you can consider some of the other sources of income that may exist but are not scheduled to pay out regularly. This can include bonds and CDs that will eventually mature and may currently provide an interest income, stocks (which may provide a current dividend income) and other securities that can be liquidated, and real estate that can be sold.

Once you've assessed the individual's income and other accessible financial resources, it's time to look at their expenses. If the patient lives in a home or receives home health care, any amount of care exceeding long-term care insurance policy limits should be added to the monthly expenses. You must also consider Medicare expenses, deductibles and the possibility the patient might enter the donut hole, a point at which Medicare prescription drug benefits stop paying until out-of-pocket expenses reach a certain amount.

A monthly budget is helpful in this situation, but it's also good to do a long-term budget so you know your monthly budget doesn't exceed their assets over the coming years. This is a complex task that generally requires the assistance of a financial planner, CPA or other professional. Some of the factors you'll need to consider include:

- The tax consequences of retirement income, liquidating assets, dividends and interest.

- Insurance policies that haven't been accessed but that could be in the future, such as life insurance with cash values or an accelerated benefit rider.

- Increases in cost of care and other expenses due to inflation.

- Inflation protection built into annuities and care policies.

- Spousal support needs. If the patient has a spouse, that individual will need a portion of the income to support their needs as well.

- Long-term care policy limits.

After establishing the patient's bills and creating a budget that works within the confines of his or her income and other financial resources, it's good to set up direct deposit into the patient's account for income and automate what bills you can. Not only will this be safer in terms of theft, but it will also create a paper trail and make financial management less stressful for you.

Planning for the Legacy

If you find, after working on the budget and evaluating the financial assets, there will likely be an inheritance when the patient passes away and there is no will or trust in place, you have some tough decisions to make. If the patient is in the early stages, you may be able to meet with an attorney and create a trust and will that spells out the patient's ultimate legacy planning desires.

If, however, the disease has progressed, there may be no option but to allow the estate to go into probate and asset distribution to be determined by the court. If you are concerned about a fair distribution that lives up to what you think your loved one would have wanted, you might meet with an elder law attorney to learn about your options.

Caregiver Legacy

As you deal with your loved one's struggle with Alzheimer's, don't forget to set up your own estate plan so your family can avoid much of the trauma and confusion caused when an individual becomes mentally incapacitated or dies without his or her wishes in writing.

The lessons in this book aren't just relevant to those suffering with Alzheimer's; they can help ensure you don't have your own legacy-planning nightmare.

Chapter 5: Pre-Need Planning

Selecting beneficiaries and weighing the possible consequences of a selection is just one step that should be taken before your death. Making and securing your post-death funeral and burial arrangements are another.

Notifying Relatives and Friends

While members of your immediate family will likely be aware of your passing, you may have distant relatives and old friends who you'd like told. Leave instructions for your family regarding how you want your other relatives and friends notified. You can also include instructions for notifying doctors, service providers, fraternal groups, schools and other relevant organizations.

The more information you leave your grieving relatives, the easier you'll make the process and the more likely it is to be done right. Consider preparing an address book with the contact information for each individual or group you want notified.

With this resource, you can also leave behind information about where to find your Last Will and Testament as well as your funeral and burial instructions. Consider also listing insurance policies charged with paying for the various services you may have had in the weeks and days before your passing, such as long-term care and medical treatment. This will allow your family to ensure all services are paid for and your legacy isn't affected.

Lastly, your family will need to notify your creditors, financial institutions, insurers and others who may continue billing you without notification of your passing. You can leave behind a copy of your monthly and annual statements and invoices so your family has a complete picture of whom they need to contact.

The Obituary

After a full life, there will be many things you'll want people to know and remember about you, and maybe some of diminished importance you don't want memorialized. If you feel the desire to completely control your printed obituary, you can write one in advance. Otherwise, you can leave notes behind about the people and accomplishments you think are most important to mention.

The Service

A funeral and memorial service may be more of a ritual to comfort the living, but they also provide an important closing ceremony on your life. If it's important to you to guide this ceremony to a large or small extent, then you should leave behind instructions for your family members to follow.

Consider every aspect of the service that's important to you, from where it's held to what scripture or poetry is read, what music or hymns are played and who should perform the service. Don't forget about other vital details such as whether it's to be an open or closed casket (or if you want your cremated remains on display), what you want to be dressed in and what jewelry you'd like to wear.

If this is difficult for you to record and you don't want to have a family member take down your instructions, consider selecting your funeral home in advance and working with them to complete a pre-need arrangement. If you do this, be certain to leave the name of the funeral home and the director who took your requests.

The Remains

Many people have very strong religious or personal feelings about how they want their remains handled after they've passed away. It's important to be very clear about how you want your remains handled when leaving behind these instructions for your family.

Check into the legality of certain wishes you may have, as well as the cost, to ensure your wishes are practical. If you want an alternative burial, such as having your cremated ashes turned into an artificial coral reef or you want an eco-friendly casket, be sure to provide your family with the information about the companies that offer these services.

Prepayment

Paying in advance for your desired service, burial, cremation or other disposal method is the best way to ensure your directives are followed and your family has less of a financial burden after your passing.

When you do prepay for your arrangements, make sure to let someone in your immediate family know and include the information, as well as the receipt, with your Last Will and Testament so your family doesn't accidentally duplicate your efforts.

Lastly, you can consider a funeral trust. Not only can this hold assets meant to pay off your funeral but the trust can also lock in current rates in order to help control costs for your heirs. As with other trusts, funeral trusts can be revocable—meaning you can revoke the trust and reassert control of the assets—or irrevocable, which means no changes can be made after the trust is formed.

Chapter 6: Worksheets

In this section, you'll have several worksheets to complete to help you determine and fine-tune your goals so you have a better understanding of how you should structure your beneficiary designations to create your ultimate legacy.

Pre- and Postdeath Assets, Income and Expenses

Worksheet A

One of the first considerations to make about your life insurance and annuity death benefits is how they might be necessary to help your family sustain your current way of life after they lose your income. Financial obligations, like income, may not remain the same after the death of one of the income-earning spouses. The sheet on the following page is a tool you can work on with your significant other to determine how either of your deaths may affect your bills and income. Completing this worksheet will give you a better idea about what you both need to leave behind.

Housing			Health Care	
Mortgage/Rent	$		Heath Insurance Premiums	$
Home Insurance	$		Prescriptions	$
Real Estate Taxes	$		Co-pays/Co-Insurance	$
Utilities	$		LTC Insurance	$
Other	$		Miscellaneous	
Living Expenses	Needs	Wants	Taxes	$
Groceries	$	$	Life Insurance Premiums	$
Clothing	$	$	Charitable Contributions	$
Auto Payments	$	$	Notes:	
Auto Insurance	$	$		
Misc. Auto Expenses	$	$		
Travel	$	$	Total Monthly Expenses: $	
Other Living Expenses	$	$		
Entertainment & Gifts	$	$		

Worksheet B

Worksheet B discusses the income your family will have after your death. Ultimately, it should leave them with enough to carry the postdeath expenses listed in the previous worksheet.

Income Sources	Estimated Monthly Income
Pension Plan	$
Social Security	$
Investments	$
Part-Time Employment	$
Other	$
B) Estimated Monthly Income	$

Total Monthly Expenses (from Worksheet A)	$
Total Estimated Monthly Income (B)	$
Postdeath Income Gap (A-B)	$

Worksheet C

Worksheet C helps you better refine your goals for your assets both before and after your death.

What are your goal(s) for your money/estate? _____

_____

_____

_____

_____

	Yes	No
Have you set up a power of attorney?		
Do you need to provide care for a child, spouse or parent after your death?		
Do you have income from real estate?		
Do you expect an inheritance that will pass through to your heirs?		
Do you have a will or a trust? Is the trust irrevocable?		
Have you planned for your burial?		
Do you have funds set aside for long-term care expenses so they won't wipe out your legacy?		

Worksheet D

Worksheet D allows you to review your current planning and identify any gaps or beneficiary appointments that could be improved. It also serves as a helpful guide to your beneficiaries when they review your assets and get a handle on your estate.

Active Policies

Company	Policy Type	Face Amount	Insured	Beneficiary

Investment/Retirement Accounts

Name/Type	Est. Value at Death	Maturity Date	Beneficiary

Other Assets

Type of Asset	Est. Value at Death	Beneficiary
Home/Rental Property		
Social Security		
Variable Annuities		
Fixed Annuities		
Total Property Value		

Contact Information

Type of Asset	Company Address and Phone Number
Home/ Property Insurance	
Annuities	
Health Insurance	
Life Insurance	
Checking Accounts	
Savings Accounts	
Retirement Accounts	
Trustee	
Attorney	

Beneficiary Designation Change

As you now know, the beneficiary designations on all your assets—from life insurance policies to annuities to 401(k)s to IRAs—are more than just instructions for the post-death distribution of your assets. They're potential tax nightmares, probate pitfalls and single-generational traps for your heirs. Ensuring your beneficiary designations are properly handled before you become seriously ill or injured is one of the best ways to make the experience less painful for your loved ones while still making certain they get the most benefit from your assets after you pass on.

You can start by keeping current all the beneficiary forms for your assets. Update your address, chosen beneficiary, contingent beneficiary or secondary benefit distribution method (such as per stirpes).

If you aren't certain who your present beneficiaries are, use the following letter template to request that information from your benefits administrator or insurance company. Remember, if you are not the owner of the policy, they may refuse to send you the information.

Beneficiary Change Letter

Company Name

Mailing Address

City, State, Zip

Attention Human Resources Department (or *Policy Services* for life insurance):

Please send me the beneficiary designation information for the following accounts:

1. Account number/policy number:

2. Account number/policy number:

3. Account number/policy number:

4. Account number/policy number:

I would like this information to include both primary and contingent beneficiary designations, percentages and policy ownership information. Please also attach a new beneficiary designation form so I may change beneficiaries if necessary.

If another individual has access to this information and it cannot be provided to me, please give me the contact information for that individual or entity.

Thank you,

_____

Pre-Needs Planning

Worksheet E

This worksheet can help you determine what steps you need to take now in order to make the postdeath process easier on your heirs.

Premade Funeral Arrangements	Yes/No	Information about Arrangements
Memorial		
Casket		
Plot		
Clothing		
Flowers		
Music		
Transportation		
Obituary		

Documents	Yes/No	Where They May Be Found*
Will		
Birth Certificate		
Life Insurance		
Medical Insurance		
Other Insurance		
Checking Account		
Savings Account		
Executor/trix		

*For the ease of your heirs, consider having all documents in one location, such as a lockbox.

ADDITIONAL BOOKS AND PROGRAMS BY DENNIS M. POSTEMA

DESIGNING YOUR LIFE

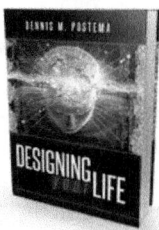

What would happen if you discovered you could do more than just live your life—you could *design* it? This book teaches you to harness the power of your subconscious and program it to help you live a happy life fitting your definition of perfection.

DESIGNING YOUR LIFE: ACTION GUIDE

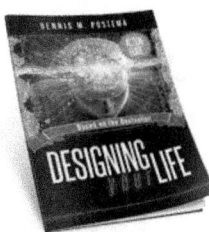

These exercises help you master your subconscious, abolish negativity and raise self-esteem. This guide focuses on creative visualization and powerful affirmations, to control your life's design and master your future.

DEVELOPING PERSEVERANCE

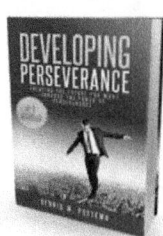

A combination of internal roadblocks are holding you back, preventing you from persevering. This book shows you how to break through these self-imposed obstacles to begin moving along your true path, taking you further than you ever thought possible.

DEVELOPING PERSEVERANCE: ACTION GUIDE

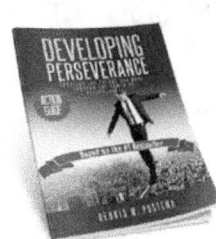

With this guide, you'll learn about the unique roadblocks you've designed for yourself and explore the thoughts, feelings and events that impact your ability to succeed.

YOU DESERVE TO BE RICH

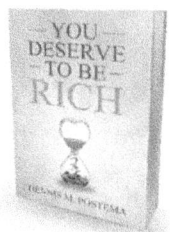

If you're busy blaming your lack of wealth on upbringing, education and environment, you're missing out on learning how easy it is to get rich. This book teaches you to throw away the excuses and focus on the 12 steps to securing a future of financial success.

YOU DESERVE TO BE RICH: ACTION GUIDE

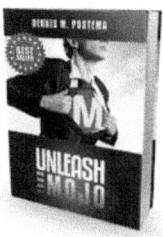

You deserve an ideal life. This workbook helps you get there by providing activities and strategies that explain the rules of greatness, help define your dreams and work to banish your fears.

UNLEASH YOUR MOJO

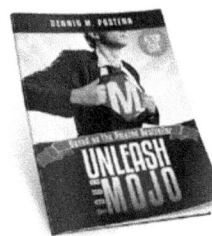

You already possess everything you need to be the person you want to be, you just have to access these powerful traits. In *Unleash Your Mojo*, you'll learn to recognize all the greatness inside you and discover how to put it to use and start living your ideal life.

UNLEASH YOUR MOJO: ACTION GUIDE

Each of us has power to succeed yet many of us never tap into that power. Instead we stagnate on the sidelines while others flash forward in life. This workbook gives practical tips, advice and exercises to advance in your quest for authenticity and power.

THE POSITIVE EDGE

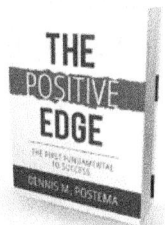

There's a secret behind living a happy, successful, fulfilling life: *Positivity.* Learn how to overcome your tendency toward negativity, how to control your life and future, and how easy it is to improve your confidence and self-esteem.

SPARK: THE KEY TO IGNITING RADICAL CHANGE IN YOUR BUSINESS

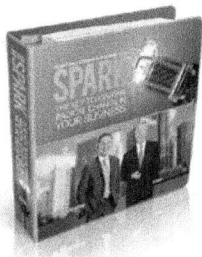

A complete, step-by-step training program to help you become a high performer and higher earner. Learn how to rise to the top of your profession, position yourself as an expert and attract the abundance you desire.

DARE TO SUCCEED

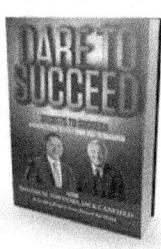

Get the motivation and the information you need to rise to the next level of success! America's #1 Success Coach, Jack Canfield, has gathered together the top business minds in one powerful book. This guide contains their secret strategies to conquer the competition and bring ongoing abundance into your life.

VICTORY JOURNAL

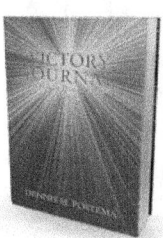

The victory journal demonstrates the importance of writing down all your daily wins. Inside you'll find exercises to help define your ideal self and create action steps to move closer to your goals.

HARNESSING THE POWER OF GRATITUDE

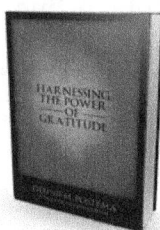

Recognize the positive energy moving through your day and harness it with this undated journal. Filled with inspirational quotes to help you maintain the spirit of gratitude, it's an ideal tool for developing an enduring, powerful habit of thankfulness.

APPRECIATING ALL THAT YOU HAVE

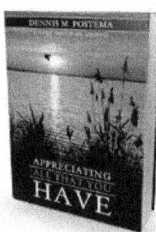

This 365-day journal filled with inspirational quotes provides a safe space to write down the many things you're thankful for. It's the perfect way to help shift your perspective and recognize the abundance of positive forces in your life.

THE PSYCHOLOGY OF SALES: FROM AVERAGE TO RAINMAKER

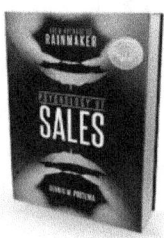

Take your sales from lackluster to rainmaker without any smarm, aggressive tactics or dishonesty. This book teaches sales pros the psychology of their customers so they can present products the right way for each shopper.

THE PSYCHOLOGY OF SALES: ACTION GUIDE

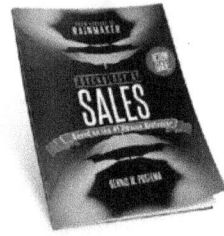

In this action guide, you'll gain greater insight into your own personality and psychological makeup as well as that of your customers so you can further your sales success and transform your career.

RETIREMENT YOU CAN'T OUTLIVE

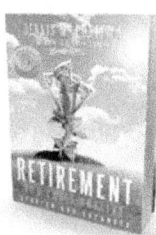

Cut through the hype and challenge conventional wisdom with a book focusing on conservative and reasonable ways to save for retirement. This book uses plain language and lots of common sense that's been missing from financial planning sessions for decades.

RETIREMENT YOU CAN'T OUTLIVE: ACTION GUIDE

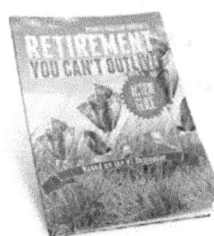

Transform the lessons taught in *Retirement You Can't Outlive* into action steps that change the shape of your financial future. This immersive tool contains worksheets, exercises and review sheets to help you develop a plan to rescue your financial future.

NAVIGATING THROUGH MEDICARE

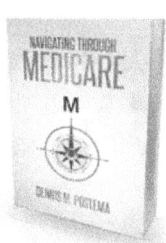

Don't be confused by the rules, plans and parts of Medicare. This book simplifies the complex system and allows you to quickly and easily make the right decision for the future of your healthcare. It's a one-stop guide to everything you need to know.

AVOIDING A LEGACY NIGHTMARE

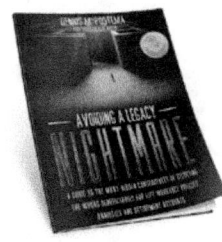

Poor planning can rip your estate from your loved ones. *Avoiding a Legacy Nightmare* is a simple guide to help you get started in creating an effective estate plan that achieves all that you intended.

PHYSICIANS: MONEY FOR LIFE

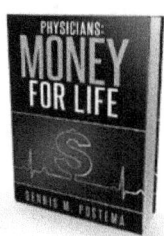

If you want to retire on your own terms, you must understand the special considerations that physicians need to make in order to maintain sustainable retirement plans. *Physicians: Money for Life* casts aside traditional advice that's not suited to conservative retirement planning and focuses on helping physicians design a plan that creates money for life.

PHYSICIANS: MONEY FOR LIFE: ACTION GUIDE

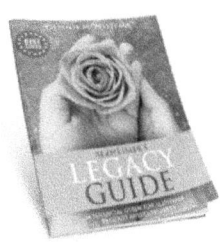

You have the knowledge necessary to change the financial health of your retirement, now it's time to apply it. This action guide helps you transform the lessons taught in *Physicians Money for Life* into action steps you can take to change the shape of your retirement. With worksheets, exercises and review, this guide will help you move forward in your retirement planning journey while devising a plan to save it.

ALZHEIMER'S LEGACY GUIDE

Alzheimer's patients and their caregivers face a race against the clock and must learn how to cement a well-thought-out legacy plan before the disease's mental, emotional and psychological effects start to take their toll. This book provides guidance to both the recently diagnosed and those who will care for them as the disease progresses.

FINANCING YOUR LIFE: THE STORY OF FOUR FAMILIES

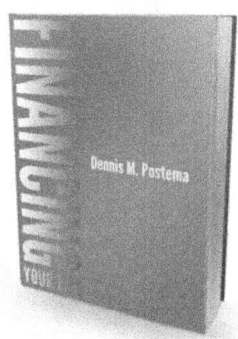

A novel that follows four families as they struggle to overcome debt, spending addiction, and unrealistic expectations in order to create financial security.

McKenna, a single mom of two boys, works hard every day as a waitress, but she can't make ends meet. When her ex-husband has an accident that prevents him from paying child support, the walls of poverty slowly close in.

Toby and Shannon, two professionals battling a layoff and personal spending demons, must find a way to work together with honesty—a proposition that's tougher than Toby expected.

Blake and Christine, a newlywed couple in a hurry to start living the good life, regardless of their ability to afford it, work together to figure out how to get the house they dream of while starting a family and battling depression.

Marcie and Kurt, two young parents struggling to keep up in an image-obsessed world, must decide whether "fitting in" is more important than financial security.

FINANCING YOUR LIFE: A GUIDE TO CONTROLLING YOUR FINANCES, TODAY

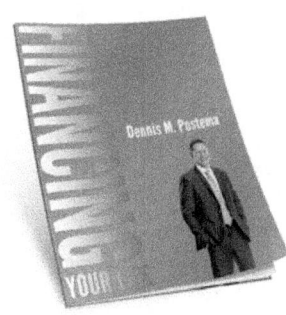

Financing Your Life is an innovative workbook devoted to teaching you how to take total control over your financial life. Within, you'll learn about the secret behind financial planning, budgeting basics, insurance, credit repair, getting out of debt, developing financial compromise with a spouse or partner, saving and investing, mortgages and more.

This tool does more than just tell you about financial concepts; it helps you begin immediately integrating what you learn into your own financial life.